EXECUTIVE MEDICINE

J. Mark Anderson, MD, DABFM
Walter Gaman, MD, DABFM, CCFP, FCP, FAAFP
with Judith Gaman, BSHS, CMA, CCRC, CAPS

TATE PUBLISHING, LLC

Published in the United States of America
by Tate Publishing, LLC
127 East Trade Center Terrace
Mustang, OK 73064
(888) 361–9473

This book is designed to provide accurate and authoritative information with regard to the subject matter covered. This information is given with the understanding that neither the author nor Tate Publishing, LLC is engaged in rendering legal, professional advice. Since the details of your situation are fact dependent, you should additionally seek the services of a competent professional.

ISBN: 1-9332908-9-7

Executive Medicine:
Optimizing Your Chances at a Longer Life

Authors:
J. Mark Anderson, MD, DABFM
Walter Gaman, MD, DABFM, CCFP, FCP, FAAFP
with
Judith Gaman, BSHS, CMA, CCRC, CAPS

DEDICATIONS

This book is dedicated to my Grandmother, who showed me that a positive attitude could help you through most anything, and my Grandfather, who knew that a little bit of bourbon prevented most everything.

J. Mark Anderson, MD, DABFM

This book is dedicated to all those patients and doctors in this hurly, burly world who want to get it right. This is for those doctors who want to master the practice of medicine and provide the best quality health care for their patients in an unhurried and comprehensive fashion. This is for those patients who realize that optimizing their health by preventing disease is priceless.

Walter Gaman, MD, DABFM,
CCFP, FCP, FAAFP

I dedicate my efforts on this publication to my mother. She has always been a great source of encouragement and has taught me that through God all things are possible. Her influence on me, even in the early years, always steered me towards the medical field and helping others.

Judith Gaman, BSHS, CMA, CCRC, CAPS

Acknowlegements

I would like to acknowledge Judy Gaman as a contributing author to this book for her tireless efforts. I want to thank Tate Publishing for their faith in our project.

Walter Gaman, MD, DABFM,
CCFP, FCP, FAAFP

We would like to thank Siemens Medical Solutions for providing an image library. A special acknowledgement goes out to Professor Paul C. Lauterbur, for allowing us to use a photo from his personal collection. We are truly honored to have cooperation from such a distinguished individual.

J. Mark Anderson, MD, DABFM
Walter Gaman, MD, DABFM, CCFP, FCP, FAAFP
Judith Gaman, BSHS, CMA, CCRC, CAPS

Table of Contents

PREFACE

Are you ready to take charge of your health? In this book, you will be given the tools to help you make positive changes to your daily routine and increase your chances at a longer, healthier life. Too many people are just playing out their lives as if they would a poker hand, just waiting for what they will be dealt. From the turn of each page, you will become educated in the mindset of executive medicine and preventative care geared toward the busy individual.

In the office, you would never dream of letting things go without checking to ensure that each department is running to par. Why then, would anyone be so lax with his or her health? Take charge and find out how each "department" in your body is running, and find ways to fine-tune them. Know the warning signs and what to do if your body is telling you that something is wrong.

Find a great physician who will take the time to listen and "serve" as your physician. Just as you hire only the top people to give you reports that you count on, so too should you hire your physician. The physician that is right for you should be in tune to your needs, and should be well versed in the field of executive health. By understanding the health risks of individuals who handle uniquely high levels of stress, such physicians can properly treat and advise such individuals.

Many doctors go through medical school thinking that he or she will solve the health problems of the world, or at least save a number of lives a day. It isn't until they are out for a few years that they decide the world is much different than they think. The problems of the world are very complex and much more involved than any course they took in medical school, and some people just choose not to be saved. There are some people that would refuse to take care of themselves even if they had all the time and resources in the world.

With that in mind, we suddenly realized that our medical careers should change focus and be geared toward those individuals who do want to take care of themselves. We want to focus on those individuals who want to eat right, stay fit, and never take a chance of losing their life to their own laziness.

If you are reading this preface, chances are that you fall into the latter category. Good for you. You should be proud, and so should your family. This tells everyone that you care not only about yourself, but them as well. This book is for you, the reason we went to medical school, the small percentage of the world that God willing, we will be able to save, at least on some level.

If you do only one thing in the next few days, complete this book. After that, follow up with a thorough physical exam that includes an executive summary and recommendations. This book is just the beginning of a more health conscious you.

INTRODUCTION

The next few pages are designed to make you think. That is why some of the chapters will seem a little technical or somewhat like a textbook. The purpose is to give you the tools that you will need to help you understand the affects of your busy schedule on your health, and when and how you should monitor those affects. The chapters are also designed to give you sound advice on many of the topics that all individuals have in common, such as stress, travel, and nutritional deficiencies.

This book starts out with a lesson in medical history. It is important to understand what drives health care today. The chapter was included with the mentality that you can never be briefed on a subject without first having a clear understanding of the historical facts.

With the changes that the world has seen, the change in the workforce has to be one of the most significant. It is not only significant on Wall Street, but in the lives and health of individuals everyday. Understanding the complexity of a stressful day, and how it affects both men and woman, will help make sense of some of the struggles we face each day. In an effort to manage stress and stressful situations, such situations must first be recognized.

Today's executive is so different in many ways from those of even ten years ago. Technology advancements have put everyone into 24/7 work mode. Between power lunches, traveling, and juggling the family, there is often nothing left to give. Being stretched too thin creates a level of mental exhaustion never before experienced.

At the end of the day, one just needs a little personal space. Some refer to it as a cave to crawl into, even if it is just a favorite chair. The pages of chapter four incorporate the needs of personal space with ideas on how to accomplish a little peace among the chaos. This chapter was written by Judy Gaman, owner of La Dame Aux Lavande Designs, and is a great argument for spending time meeting your personal space needs in an effort to increase your efficiency and effectiveness.

In the final chapters of this book, you will learn how to track family medical history and make commitments and concessions for your own preventative health. You will obtain a broad understanding of the executive physical, and how it differs from what many refer to as a routine physical exam. Also, you will be informed of how to keep records and when to update information. Proper documentation of your health history is essential.

Maybe one of the most important chapters of the book, *Defining 100%,* will give you the tools you need to stop running the rat race and start giving 100% to everyone, including yourself. By setting priorities and managing those priorities, life will become enjoyable again.

Last of all, a word about *Tying it All Together:* taking all the things this book has taught and bringing it together in a way that helps you apply it. You are in charge of your health, and you are responsible for your preventative care. Take charge now by reading this book in its entirety and then applying what you have learned today, not tomorrow.

Great thought has been put into what contents should be on the following pages. Determining what information is pertinent to changing your lifestyle in a positive way is interjected with sound medical facts that help drive home the message. Taking care of your best asset–your health–will enhance your ability to enjoy life, work smarter, and plan for a bright future.

Chapter One

The History of Medicine

In the business world, we understand companies by first learning about their past, then their current status, and eventually their projected future. In medicine, most people look to the present and the future, but pay little attention to the past, regardless of its impact on today. This first chapter is designed to help you understand the advancements of medicine and how those advancements can help forecast a bright future for your chances at a healthier life.

Over the past one hundred years, the life expectancy rates have increased; whereas, the average person lived to be just over 47 years old in 1900, the average age was 77 in 2001. This increase is phenomenal, and people are now living the equivalency of almost two lives, which is mostly due to advancements in medicine. The largest increase rate occurred in the first fifty years of the 1900s. In fact, the average expectancy increased by 21 years between 1900 and 1950, which coincided with the timing of many significant medical advancements, such as the discovery and production of penicillin.

In 2002, United States governmental statistics showed that the leading causes of death in persons over 50 were cancers and circulatory system failures. Therefore, it is no surprise that people over the age of 50 are more likely to have significantly more years added to their life expectancy than they were just 10 years ago. The medical imaging advancements for detecting cancer and heart problems are extraordinary. Such advancements are creating opportunity for early detection and intervention. What does all this mean to you, the busy executive? It means the opportunity to enjoy life after retirement, to spend time with your significant other on islands off the Caribbean, or to take up that hobby that you never had time to do.

Medicine has come a long way, and many advancements have been made that allow us to enjoy a much healthier lifestyle. In 1927, the leading cause of death was cancer, closely followed by influenza and pneumonia. It is hard to imagine now, but people did die from the flu. A pandemic of influenza actually killed 600,000 US citizens from 1918–1919. Now, in our quick-fix society, you can stop by your physician's office or a participating pharmacy and receive a flu vaccine for a nominal fee. In late 2004, the FDA halted a large number of the vaccinations for influenza. This recall alarmed many health professionals who understood the possible ramifications. All too often we forget about the past and take things such as a vaccination for granted.

Vaccinations have been responsible for stopping and preventing serious outbreaks such as polio, pneumonia, and many others. These preventative measures, coupled with treatments such as antibiotics and antivirals, have not permitted many of the health risks that were once so feared to be anything more than a mere interruption to our schedules.

Technology has made miraculous strides in developing the tools physicians need in making a proper diagnosis. It is hard to believe that Professor Paul Lauterbur and Professor Mansfield, developed the Magnetic Resonance Imaging (MRI) such a short time ago, and it in 1980 it became commercially available. This was preceded by the invention of the Computed Tomography (CT) scanner in 1972 by Godfrey Hounsfield of EMI Laboratories, and Allan Cormack of Tufts University, Massachusetts. MRI and CT are now used routinely and have been credited with saving millions of lives through early detection and intervention.

In 1986, the Human Genome Initiative began. Over a 13-year span, the Initiative has had a reported $3 billion spent on its progress. The research on human genetics has brought forth a new understanding of many of the diseases and disorders that plague the human race. The fascination of DNA research has caught the attention of many of the world's greatest scientists and, the project has gained worldly attention. New strides have been made in understanding the role our genetic make-up has in determining our destiny. Not only has genetic research been able to determine the risks for diseases such as Alzheimer's, but new genetic studies have linked stress to DNA damage that leads to cancers and cardiac problems.

The discoveries in genetics have not only given us a look into ourselves as humans, but they have made way for unsurpassed medical advancements. The study of pharmacogentics/parmacogenomics will soon find common place among all clinical advancements and clinical trials. As the genetic research continues, it makes finding links between genetic factors and drug efficacy much easier. These studies will yield an easier way for physicians to prescribe medications in the right class and right dose based on the individual needs of the patient. This research could also help prevent foreseen side effects in sub-populations that are not ideal matches for a particular treatment.

These are exciting times for our generation to be living, with the possibility of long lives filled with many active years. We should all be thankful to the men and women who have devoted their lives and careers to the advancement of medicine. It is time to take those advancements and apply them to our lives, to ensure the best chances of longevity.

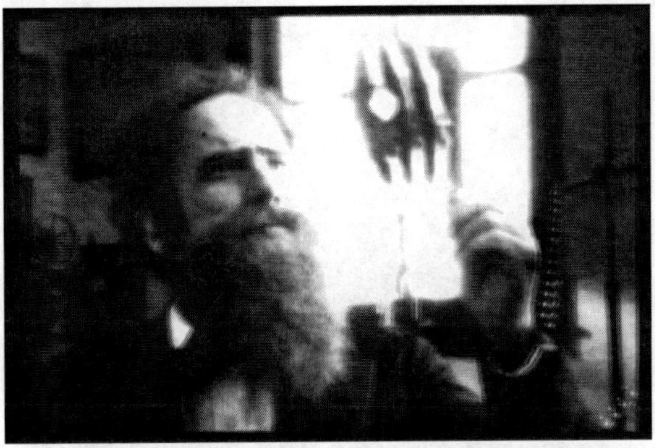

Wilhelm Conrad Röntgen
took the first x-ray on November 8, 1895.

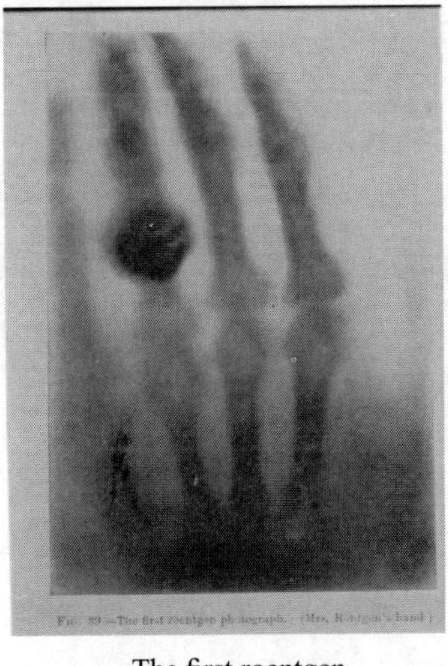

The first roentgen
photograph, or x-ray, was of Mrs.
Rontgen's hand. Author: Glasser, Otto.
National Library of Medicine

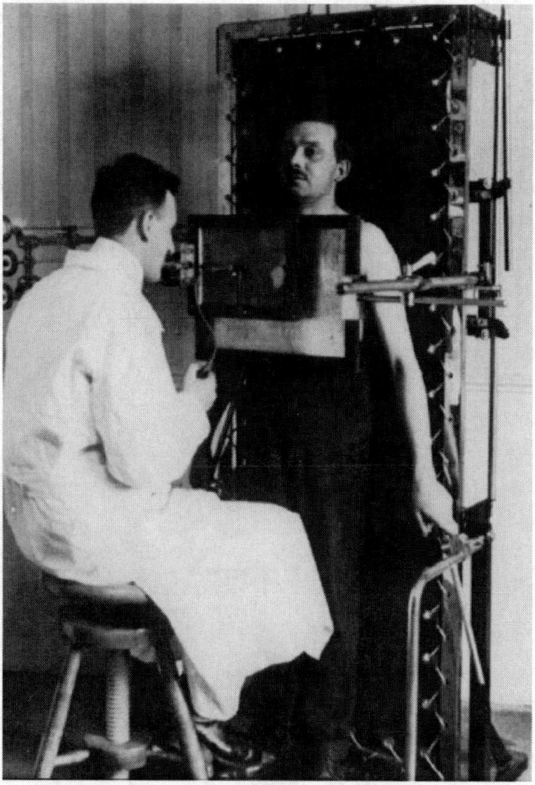

Early x-ray system 1907, Klinoscop. Photo courtesy of Siemens Medical Solutions.

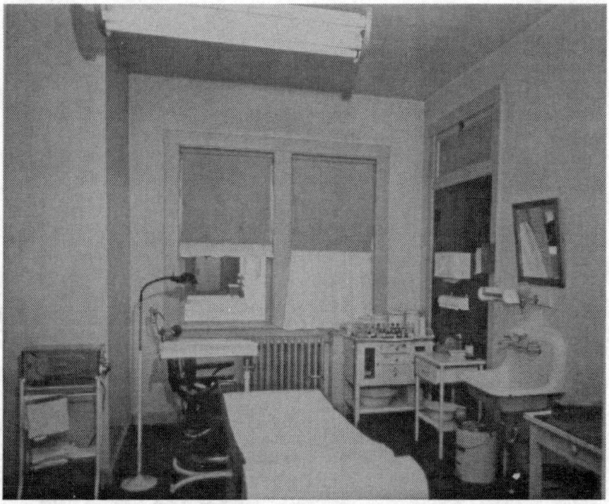

Early exam rooms were cold and uninviting.
National Library of Medicine.

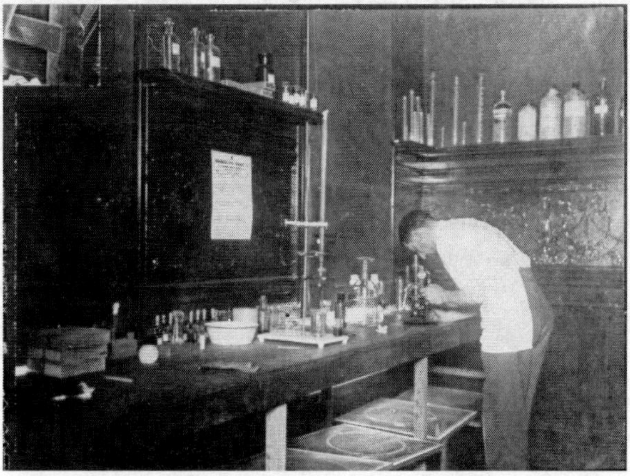

Microscopes provided a glimpse into the future of modern medicine. This photo is from San Francisco, CA and was taken in 1908. National Library of Medicine.

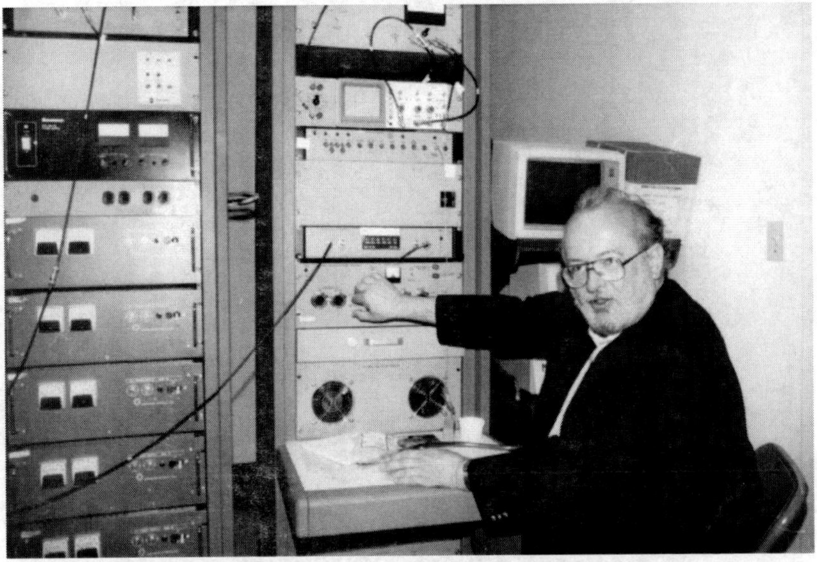

Paul C. Lauterbur, who was involved in inventing MRI is shown here in the late 1970's. The MRI not only excels at diagnosing disease, but often reveals the actual nature of disease and injuries, helping doctors avoid inappropriate surgery and medications. Professor Lauterbur received the Nobel Prize 2003 for Physiology or Medicine (jointly with Sir Peter Mansfield).
Photo courtesy of Professor Lauterbur's personal collection.

Chapter Two

History of the Working Man And the Addition of the Working Woman

Over the years, the American workforce has changed in the way it is comprised and in its complexity. It is important to understand how we arrived at this point as a country, and what you can do to ensure your executive lifestyle does not get the best of you.

From the Fields to the Corner Office

In the 1800s and early 1900s, most of the country worked on farms and produced their own food source. There was a definite division of income levels, and although by 1929, the top 5% of corporations controlled 85% of all corporate income, most people of all income classes respected the businessperson. Perhaps their respect grew from a well-known book written by Bruce Barton in 1925, entitled "*The Man*

Nobody Knows." Mr. Barton, a well-respected advertising executive, compared a business executive to Jesus, and the management team to his apostles. The book became a best seller at a time when the workforce was facing some significant changes, and catapulted the businessman into the limelight.

By the late 20s, the majority of households in America had electricity, and some began to enjoy the better things in life, such as vacuum cleaners and toasters. The National Association of Manufacturers and others associated with them began to recognize the need to offer benefit packages to employees. In an effort to increase job satisfaction, without the use of unions, who were at times the cause of employee/employer turmoil, employers started some of the first "perks" for workers.

Urbanization became the majority's choice by 1920, with 51% choosing to live in more populated areas. This percentage continued to rise to 56% by 1930. In the 1950s, suburban areas became popular with the increase in transportation availability. William Levitt became known for his "Levittown" development on Long Island, which some believe sparked the growth of suburban life and track homes. By the 1960s, the movement of the population into urban and suburban lifestyles proved to mimic the change in the labor force, as white-collar workers outnumbered the blue-collar workers. Corporations of more than 500 employees were now home to 38% of the workforce.

Changes in Physical Activity for Workers

Long gone are the days of manual labor for the majority of workers. Now, most employees sit behind a desk and work from their computers. The change from manual labor to sedentary desk jobs has played a large role in the deterioration of the health of many executives. Inactivity can lead to numerous health problems, including obesity, heart trouble, and circulation problems. Airplane travel can cause dehydration, fatigue, jet lag, extremity swelling, and a number of other symptoms. Traveling for extended periods only compounds the problems. Our bodies are on the go, and relaxation and fresh air are not usually on the agenda of most business trips.

Computers, laptops, and hand held PDAs may be convenient and necessary, but they also come with their own risks. The American Optometric Association recognizes Computer Vision Syndrome (CVS) as a common disorder among 90% of people who use the computer in excess of 3 hours per day. CVS symptoms include headache, loss of focus, and burning or tired eyes. Since most executives have constant use of some sort of computer, they are at high risk for developing CVS.

Having conveniences such as computers, personal assistants, and the best parking places may seem like great perks, but they could actually be harmful to your health, since they decrease your requirements for physical activity. Sedentary lifestyles are associated with cancer, heart disease, diabetes, dcpression, and a long list of other disorders. It is very important that you, the executive, take strides each day to increase your activity level. Taking a break from the desk every few hours and walking for 15 minutes will help with circulation and may also improve energy levels. This is a great way to decrease stress levels within the body and help even out mood throughout the day. Make sure that your walk is paced and does not include stopping and chatting along the way, or you may defeat the purpose.

Regular exercise at least three times a week is also extremely important to the health and wellness of executives, especially when the job is excessively demanding and mentally overtaxing. The old term "go out back and chop wood" was used to describe how people would deal with stress. Our ancestors had a good thing going, and we may all benefit from having a wood chopping room next to the boardroom. However, if you do not have access to one, a treadmill will do.

Exercise does not only relieve stress, it also helps to burn fat and reduces the waistline. Over time, sedentary desk jobs and power lunches will take their toll on the body, and exercise is the best weapon of defense. Keeping your weight down and your body fat percentage below 22% will increase your chances of living a longer, healthier life. Exercise will also help with the mood swings and temper problems that so many top executives tend to possess, due to their Type A personalities. If you are a Type A, do yourself and those around you a favor and go to the gym to work out your frustrations.

From the Home to the Office for Females

Women are finding themselves more involved in the corporate world, with more options for career advancement. World War II was a great turning point for women, because they were called to duty by their country, and they found themselves working to replace the many men at war. The saying that "you can never go back" holds true for the movement of women into the workforce. The employment of women rose, and in 1965, 37% of all women over sixteen were employed, followed by 50% in 1978.

Now we see many women who are working in top executive positions at major corporations. The stress and added responsibility of a working woman, especially if she is also a mother and wife, takes on a whole new health perspective. As mentioned in the previous section, there are the obvious stressors that today's executive faces. However, women face some even more difficult, and often ignored, problems that add to their stress level and cause health deterioration.

Just for a moment, let's focus on a woman's feet. It really doesn't make sense to expect a woman to wear high heels all day; would a man be able to walk on his tip toes from 9–5? If he did, I bet he would take the next day off to rest (or buy new footwear). The feet are the endpoint for many nerves, and tired feet can lead to multiple health problems, such as back pain and headaches. Mainstream society and medicine have begun to recognize the importance of the feet, with reflexology finding commonplace in spas and physical therapy departments. Female executives should invest in good footwear and not be afraid to spend more money on shoes that were meant for 8–10 hour days.

Feet are important, but many women may say there are other obstacles to worry about in the corporate world. Although women face many challenges in the management positions of white collar America, one of the toughest has to be the balancing act of being a working mother and/or working wife. This can cause what we have termed Long Day Syndrome (LDS), fatigue and depression caused by adding work at home after work at the office. The social pressures on working mothers and wives to keep up the domestic pace of stay at home mothers and wives is enormous. Following the exhaustion is often a heavy dose of self-induced "PTA/PTO absentee guilt." Finding a balance of both work and home activities is important; and setting reasonable goals for that balance is the key to emotional stability. One cure of LDS is to incorporate those at home into the daily chore routines, and understand that you cannot and should not do it all.

TIPS for the Executive

A few things that can ease the pain of a long day at the office:

• Drink at least two 8 oz. glasses of water

• Take breaks from the desk and go for short walks

• Stretch every hour to increase blood flow and stimulate hormone release

• Smile and think yourself happy (this really can work)

• Have proper footwear (both men and women)

• Look away from your computer every 10 minutes and focus on the wall for at least 15 seconds to give your eyes a rest and prevent eye strain

• If traveling, take a walk in the fresh air during meeting breaks

Chapter Three

Today's Executive

There is no such thing as banker's hours any longer. In the past, people in "office clothes," although respected, were often teased about the lack of hours or effort that went into a full days work. The tables have turned; the average executive or businessperson puts in many hours of overtime and often works to the point of mental exhaustion. In the world of executives, there are no time clocks to punch and no one to take over on the next shift. Instead, all the deadlines rest on the shoulders of the person responsible for meeting them. These deadlines sometimes overpower the important things in life, such as family, relaxation, and mealtime, resulting in an unbalanced and overstressed human being. This is not exactly what was intended for the human race.

Power Lunches

Somewhere in time, it not only became acceptable to work through lunch, but it became fashionable. Power lunches, networking lunches, and lunch meetings are all too common in the work place. Our society thinks that stopping to eat a meal without distraction is simply a waste of good time. This way of thinking is social injustice to the digestive tract!

From a medical standpoint, multiple lunch meetings are unhealthy and a bad habit to fall into. The occasional meeting is ok, but getting into a daily routine of "eating while meeting" is dangerous. First, the lunch hour should be reserved for a break from the daily stress, a moment of reflection and enjoyment. It should also be a time when you can take in food, hopefully healthy, and digest it properly. In order to do so, you must chew properly and eat at a rate comparable to your digestive system. Gulping down a big lunch without an ounce of relaxation is a perfect prescription for developing digestive disorders, such as ulcers and acid reflux.

You can avoid lunch hour meetings by simply refusing to have more than one a month, or if you are extremely pressed, no more than one a week. During your crunch lunch, order light and be sure to slow down and chew properly. If you anticipate the meeting to be especially stressful, choose low fat and low carbohydrate foods (the opposite of what you will crave). Remember that you are in charge of your time and your health.

Travel, Travel, Travel

According to recent United States Bureau of

Transportation Statistics, an estimated 399 million long-distance trips in the US are related to business each year. This means nights away from home, many times cramped for hours in a hotel. If you are like most executives, this also paints a picture of a mini-bar raid for nuts and a beer during the wee hours of the night. Do yourself a favor and don't make this a habit.

Traveling for long hours, whether in a car or an airplane, decreases circulation and causes fluid retention. If you travel often, this could cause long lasting damage to your circulatory system. Keep track of the hours you have been sitting and try to exercise for at least 10 minutes for every hour that you have been sedentary. For example, if you have a four-hour flight, hit the hotel gym for at least 40 minutes to relieve tension and increase circulation. The 10:1 ratio will also help reduce fatigue common with travel, as well as reduce mental stress associated with your trip.

Technology is advancing, and the world is becoming more and more adaptive to a global work environment. Everywhere you turn, you have the option to get a little more work done. Cell phones, lap tops, temporary internet connections and more have all but turned us into robots. Do not get into the trap of "have lap-top and cell phone, will travel 24/7" or you will soon be in the business of "have coffin, will travel–one-way." Take time to see, hear, and smell your surroundings. Stop arriving and wondering how you got there; instead, take time to live in the moment and for the moment whenever possible.

You may be able to mentally remove yourself from the conscious state of "work" and bring yourself back to the here and now. If this does not come easy to you, sign up for meditation classes or attend a seminar on relaxation. Learning how to shut your brain down for a few moments will keep you from reaching overload. This process, we refer to as "resetting your brain," is quite helpful in reducing stress and clearing the mental junk from the corners of your mind. This is similar to shutting down and restarting a computer in order for it to run more efficiently.

In addition to exercise and relaxation, it is important to follow a healthy diet and drink plenty of water. Water is very important to the proper function of the body, and proper hydration is a requirement for healthy traveling. Some people find drinking bottled water to be an easier way of keeping track of their intake.

The bottom line for traveling is to take extra notice of your actions during a trip. Remember that your body is under the stress of traveling and needs a little extra attention. Business trips should not be a signal to work 14-hour days, and if your days do become long and tedious, take the time to relax and remember that you are human.

Juggling Act

As much as we would all like to think that

things are always peachy at home and at the office, it is just not reality. Chances are you are running around juggling the job, kids, and home responsibilities as best you can. Between soccer practices, piano lessons, a date with your spouse, and that report that is due–there is not much time for you. Finding a way to organize the chaos is not a luxury, it is a necessity.

Each day seems to run into the next, weeks into months, months into years. Take the time to set your priorities and be loyal to them. If you are too tired to go to church with your family, stop staying up so late, or arrange your travel so that you are home from your trips earlier. If you have neglected a "date-night" with your spouse, put it on the calendar and make it a priority. Date nights are much cheaper than a divorce, and proper communication between you and your spouse is vital to a healthy relationship. Besides, you may just remember what attracted you to them in the first place. Every family should have a family calendar. These are usually quite large and find their home on the refrigerator door. Give each person a different color marker and log his or her schedule in their color. Family events should be logged in black. This will allow each person to see the "big picture" for each day. Although this seems like a simple task, it is vital to becoming organized.

Here are a few tips on how to make your life easier.

• Join a car pool for children's sport practices

• Choose a dry cleaner that picks up and delivers

• Hire a housekeeper and have them also do laundry

• Give the kids chores!

• Schedule time for you, and ensure that your spouse has some personal time as well

• Eat at least 3 meals a week at the family table, especially if you have kids (Every Dinner is preferable, but may not fit your travel schedule)

• Make a point of saying at least one good thing to one person each day

• If you have a lawn, hire a lawn service (you can still plant flowers if you enjoy yard work)

• Meditate or spend time in prayer every day

• Always keep healthy snacks in the kitchen to avoid binge eating before bed

• Be your own personal boss (your attitude and health is your responsibility)

• A busy lifestyle is not necessarily a healthy one. Learn to say no to things that take up precious time that could be spent with your family and optimizing your professional duties. If you overload your plate with committees, volunteering, more projects at work, etc., you will become the Jack or Jill of all trades, but master of none. Life should be about balance, and finding the right balance is crucial to optimizing your chances for a longer life.

Unfortunately, this is how many executives would graph their time. An unbalanced life can add to stress, depression and a multitude of other health problems.

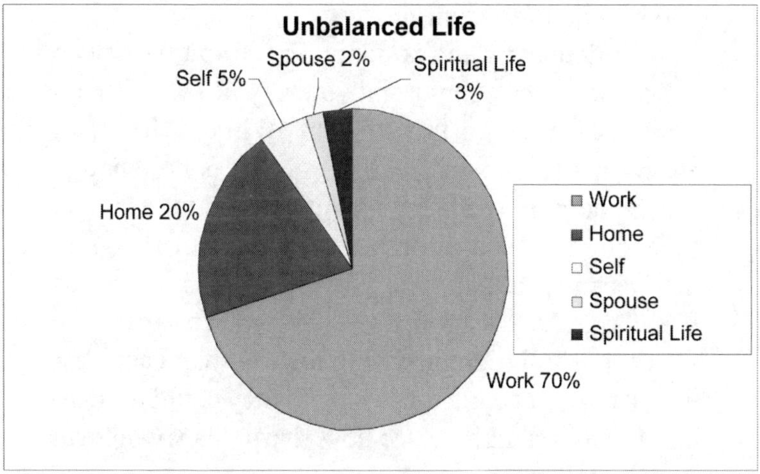

Importance of Efficiency and Mental Capacity

In the class room of a fifth grade teacher, a sign hangs that says, "If you do not have enough time to do it right, you must have enough time to do it over;

because if it is not done right, you WILL be doing it over." This principle not only applies to school aged children, but also applies to almost everything in life. Therefore, it is so important that your efficiency and accuracy levels are as high as possible, because both are equally important.

Having a lifestyle, fitness, and nutritional assessment during your executive physical is a good way to summarize what you are doing right, and what you could improve upon. Your brain cannot possibly be in great shape when the rest of your body is not. Taking care of your body as a whole is an important and basic requirement for success.

Adequate sleep is defined as 8 hours of sleep per night. Some people, and you may be one of them, think that 6 hours is sufficient. While 6 hours of sleep may leave you feeling rested, it is not enough for the body to recuperate and the brain to recharge. Sleep should be a priority on your list of things to do. Recently, a man who turned 100, celebrated his birthday with his brothers. They reported that they all sleep a full night and took an hour nap each day, which they had done for as long as they could remember. It was a delight to see how sharp this *young* man was at age 100.

There are some tricks to getting a good night sleep, especially if you have a type A personality and have trouble turning your thoughts off. One trick is to make a list of what you have to do the next day, along with any important things you want to be sure to remember. The list will reassure you that tomorrow is another day, and things can be accomplished then. Another trick is to take a warm bath and have a light healthy snack. The bath will relax you, and the snack will keep you from waking up hungry. If you are trying to loose weight, skip the snack or have it at least 3 hours before bed.

Sleeping pills are always the last resort, and any alternative is better than getting into an addictive habit that can ultimately reduce your mental awareness. Some people laugh at the warm milk advice, but it is a fact that warm milk actually causes the brain to go into relaxation and sleep mode. Tuna and dark meat turkey also have the same sleeping aid properties.

Still can't sleep? Is your mattress comfortable and your pillow the right thickness? If the answer is no, you must invest in proper sleeping materials. Take the time to shop out the right mattress, bedding, and pillow. If you have allergies, you may want to resist feather and down materials, whereas they may cause a stuffy nose and restless sleep.

Often, people have adequate sleep hours but still feel tired and mentally drained. If you experience this, especially if you snore at night, you may need a sleep study. Sleep studies are a great way to diagnose sleep apnea, a condition in which a person stops breathing during the night. The word "apnea" is from Greek origin, and actually translates to "without breath." Sleep apnea is a serious condition and is very common, but often undiagnosed. Although this condition can strike anyone, it is most common in males over 40 years of age that are somewhat overweight. If left untreated, serious side effects can occur. Sleep apnea can cause high blood pressure, weight gain, heart disease, memory loss, headaches, and even impotence. Depending on the cause of sleep apnea, different treatment options exist.

Stress and the Executive

All people experience stress at some level, and in varying degrees. Executives are unique in that they experience stress in moderate to high levels for extended periods. Meeting deadlines, making important decisions, and carrying the weight of a company on their shoulders only adds to the stress of other daily responsibilities. For most of us, there is no time to feel sorry for ourselves or just give in. Instead, it is a constant steady stream of an exhaustive to work, home, and back to work schedule.

Research over the past few years has lead to conclusions that stress can actually have a negative effect on the body and be biologically destructive. Free radicals, chemicals found in the body, are unpaired and electrically charged. Because they are unpaired and non-selective, they choose to attack anything around them and steal the charge. This creates a chain reaction, making the once healthy molecule a free radical. When levels of stress are heightened, a process called oxidative stress worsens, and the free radicals continue targeting proteins, DNA, and other important molecules. Oxidative stress has been linked to premature aging, hypertension, and many other problems. The body actually begins to deteriorate if steps are not taken to prevent the process.

Prevention begins with a comprehensive physical exam that will determine your levels of stress and overall health risks. Another, and more inclusive, way to access oxidative stress is through a genetic screening for free radical scavengers. These scavengers can be higher or lower in some individuals, and make the ability to fight off free radicals either harder or easier. To find out if you are at risk for oxidative stress, a genetic test for Oxidative Stress–1 (OS-1) can check for Superoxide Dismutase (SOD). SOD is an enzyme in the body that protects against radiation and rids the body of Super Oxides. Another test, Oxidative Stress–2 (OS- 2), tests for Glutathione Peridase (GPX). GPX detoxifies hydrogen peroxide, which can have damaging effects on protein, DNA, and lipids. These tests are not readily available at all doctor's offices, you may need to go to a clinic that specializes in executive medicine or genetic testing.

CHAPTER FOUR

CREATING YOUR PERSONAL SPACE

This chapter refers to the importance of personal space, and how your environment affects your attitude, productivity, and health. Many times this topic is ignored or deemed trivial, when indeed it is very significant. Taking time to identify your interests and create personal space can help you have a sense of identity and pride in who you are, and why you chose to stay in the surroundings that you do.

Paying Attention to Color

Although everyone is different, colors can have a definite affect on mood and creativity. For many people, the color gray can cause a feeling of depression. Many people only notice this when they live in or travel to a gloomy city, but the same problem can happen when they work or live within four gray walls. Just as interesting is the problem that white causes for many people. White has been known to cause anxiety in some, while representing cleanliness in others. Red, a color that is becoming more common in decorating, is known to arouse feelings of anger or overexcitement; while earth tones may sooth and reduce tension. Choosing colors that are right for you is an important step in creating your personal space.

The colors and effects listed above are not necessarily applicable to everyone, so you must find what colors evoke what emotions in you. An easy test for this is to obtain a color pallet and to write what comes immediately to mind when viewing each color. Pay special attention to the memories or emotions attached to each color. This will help you identify what colors are right for you and your personal spaces. When choosing your workspace colors, look for those that relax, as well as promote creativity and increased thought processes. When choosing the colors for your home, look to those that evoke emotions of happiness and a love of life. Try to keep your color choices for home and office separate, so that you will not be distracted and reminded of the other.

Simple Ways to Reduce Stress through Ambiance

The chaos of everyday life, both at home and in the office, can become overwhelming. This is why it is important to incorporate some simple aspects of decorating that will increase your ambiance, while decreasing your stress level. Finding ways to stay anchored in who you are and the things you like will help you live in the moment. Staying focused will help you make decisions that are consistent with your beliefs, and not just the outside pressures you encounter.

One way to create an ambiance is to incorporate things about you, such as your hobbies, pictures of your favorite Kodak® moments, framed poems that you find inspirational, or objects that represent your favorite childhood memories. Other ideas, such as incorporating nature through the use of fountains and other décor, may help bring the outdoors in. Careful consideration when choosing the interior design and décor of your home or office will yield great long term benefits.

Take a moment to identify the things in your personal spaces that you like and dislike. Is your chair comfortable? Do you have plain white walls that lack art? Do you need a 'Do Not Disturb' sign for your door? Should you add a little life with live plants? Take time to look around and make improvements to your space. The time spent will more than be made up for in increased comfort and productivity. If needed, hire a professional designer/decorator who understands personal space and the executive lifestyle.

Functioning in a More Efficient Workspace

Once you have created a more harmonious workspace, it is time to assess its efficiency. Make sure that you have ample file space, desk space, and that all the things that you will need in a days work are close by. Creating a balance of efficiency, while rejecting the notion of clutter, can be quite the task. Although things should be accessible, make sure that they are not distracting or taking up needed desk space. Having adequate storage and organizational tools will allow you to file items in an effective manner, and prevent the loss of important objects or documents.

Just as this is important for your space as the executive, it is equally important to those you employ. Lets face it, when they do their work more efficiently, so can you. If you have no knowledge of how to organize workspace, delegate to someone who does, or hire a professional who specializes in workspace organization and productivity acceleration. Be careful that whoever takes on the task of creating an efficient workspace does so without ruining the ambiance, which is so desperately needed to create and maintain healthy levels of cooperation and basic "good vibes" within your department or organization.

Feng Shui for the Executive Office or Home. Do the Chinese Have Something?

The American way of life has become filled with instant gratification, quick decision-making, and less and less personal and professional accountability. Our world has become inundated with unnecessary clutter and confusion, causing a country that has a majority of the population fitting into the model for attention deficit disorder. Are we clinically hyperactive? Or is it environmental pressures, most of which are self-imposed?

The Chinese have an ancient art of organizing their lives and their environment called Feng Shui (pronounced fung shway). There are many schools of thought in Feng Shui, but all incorporate the importance of harmony and flow. These Chinese concepts are a matter of common sense. Executives and all those with busy lives could benefit from incorporating such basic concepts into their daily life.

Businesses around the world rely on Feng Shui experts to help them design their company's workspace. Working spaces that flow promote cooperation among employees, increased productivity, and positive energy within the company. This book is not meant to imply that you should rush out and hire a Feng Shui expert to redesign your business and home; but we are suggesting that there are a few basic concepts that can influence your daily life.

One of the most basic and applicable concepts in Feng Shui is the reduction of clutter in your home and work life. Clutter can compile in many different forms, including physical clutter, mental clutter, and distracting clutter. Reducing clutter in your world will allow you to think more clearly, perform better, and reduce overall stress at both home and work. This is not just Feng Shui, it is basic common sense. As stated earlier, many concepts of the ancient Chinese art are common sense that we sometimes chose to ignore.

For the purpose of this chapter, we will focus on the reduction of clutter. First, physical clutter will be addressed, since it is the most obvious. Physical clutter can be defined as objects that obstruct your clear view of your life, its meaning, and the task at hand. This type of clutter can be found in your home as well as your office, and should be avoided. Look at your office. Is it filled with loose papers or stacks of things to do? If you are like most people, this type of clutter is just considered a part of the everyday hassles of life. Placing only the task at hand on your desk will help you to think more clearly, and complete the task at hand in a more efficient manner. Other tasks, not currently being completed, should be stored in organized folders and brought out when there is designated time to work on them.

Physical clutter at home can also be a problem. Is your house cluttered with toys, incomplete projects, or last weekend's left over mess? Keeping a clean and organized home will help reduce stress and promote relaxation. Whether you are married, have kids, or live alone, the person responsible for the mess should be the one to clean it up. Why is it that many executives, both male and female, hold those in the office responsible for even the littlest of things, but cannot delegate a single task at home? Delegation is not only a more peaceful way of living in harmony, but also a necessary process to ensure that the home is not chaotic and interruptive of positive energy. Take charge of your home and clean it on a regular basis. Everyone learned to clean up after himself or herself when they went through grade school, yet as adults we seem to be rebellious when it comes to keeping our own area clean. The irony is that the only people harmed by a messy house are those who live in it, including you!

Although keeping your work and life clear of physical clutter is necessary, it is only the start of creating harmony in your personal world. Mental clutter can be physically and mentally draining, as well as have serious health repercussions. Keeping things in memory that no longer serve a purpose can create a fog over the real tasks at hand. How many of your thoughts per day consists of the woulda, coulda, shoulda trilogy? Stop looking back on things of which you have no control. Learn from your mistakes and move on. Not doing so can create a paralyzing effect and damage your health, attitude, and ultimately your personal and professional future.

If you have trouble letting go, you can create a list of things that you have been holding on to and storing in your mental baggage file. After creating the list, burn it, (safely of course) and move on. Getting back to Chinese concepts, look around and identify objects that remind you of those mentally destructive thoughts. Take time to permanently remove them. An example of such objects is a gift from an ex-spouse or ex-employee that you no longer wish to expend your mental energy on.

Once you have completed the first two steps

of cleaning up your act, you can move on to the clutter that causes distraction. One of the worst terms ever coined was "multi-tasking." This term changed the way of American life. It changed the way we do everything, as well as how we view our productivity levels at home and at work. We, as a society, have also begun to create a mental competition of who can get the most done in one day. Taking time to think and reflect has almost become a thing of the past. Our computers must be faster, our television sets must have unlimited options for our viewing pleasure, and some of our favorite coffee houses are succumbing to the drive-through craze. Faster, better, more, all day long! When was the last time we analyzed faster to see if it was actually faster in the end, or better to see if it really is an improvement, or just another choice? When is the last time we just enjoyed something for what it is? A recent ad in a travel magazine boasted of a new company that can help you connect with new people. The advertisement actually stated that you could "outsource your social life" to them. It seems as though the distractions of people's everyday life are overtaking their ability to have fun and seek out others with similar interests.

Getting rid of distraction is easy, but may be a little hard to accept at first, because you are actually retraining your brain to think and not just react. Turning off the background music or the television while concentrating on your present situation can help you live in the present, and live life more fully. Learning to listen to people and absorb what they say the first time, without asking them to repeat themselves, will not only save you time, but will help earn respect from the person you are communicating with. Respect from your professional colleagues and family is something that is earned, not just assumed. Communication breakdown at home and at work are many times due to the lack of concentration and engagement by those involved. All too many times, we are thinking of something else or thinking of our response prior to even hearing the question. Make a point of listening and giving undivided attention to those around you, and you will be amazed at how your relationships will improve.

The answer to the question of this section is yes. The Chinese do have some of the answers in Feng Shui. Creating peace and harmony in your environment will improve your clarity and functionality, as well as restore peace to your life. For more information on this topic, please refer to the many books written on the topic, or to companies specializing in the ancient Chinese art.

CHAPTER 5

FAMILY HISTORY

As we learn more about the importance of our family medical history, we are able to detect and prevent diseases that our bodies may be more susceptible to. Scientists have been busy at work mapping out the genetic links to many diseases and disorders that affect all of us, either directly or indirectly. Finding ways to take good care of our bodies includes the task of identifying risks and taking measures to protect our health.

Knowing Your Family History

At the risk of sounding like a veterinarian, it is very important to identify the factors that make up your pedigree. In the world of genetic testing, they actually refer to familial disorders as part of a human pedigree. It is more important than ever to keep good family medical history records. You can first start by listing yourself and your siblings, then travel the family tree and log your parents and grandparents. If you do not know this information and it is not readily available through dictation by a relative, you may want to check death records.

The Significance of Maternal and Paternal Genetic Predispositions

It is important to know your family history and report it to your physician, so that they are able to determine what preventative measures should be taken to identify the disease or disorder, or how to prevent it from becoming fully developed in your system. Inheriting certain diseases depends on the type of pattern that is necessary for development. In some cases, it takes two gene mutations (both parents) to pass on a trait. Such a pattern is termed autosomal recessive. In the case of autosomal dominate mutations, it takes only one parent to pass on the disease or disorder. Another type, x-linked mutations, the mutation is carried on the X chromosome. In this situation, a son is more susceptible to the disorder because he only has one x chromosome, whereas a female has two, and the other may be without mutation. In the case of the female, both x chromosomes must carry the mutation. Lastly, there is another form of inherited mutations that is carried through a cell's mitochondria. The mother's egg contains mitochondria, but not the sperm; therefore, these mutations are only passed from mother to child.

Understanding the pathways of genetic disorders helps to explain the significance of family history when determining your preventative care. If you have a genetic predisposition to a particular mutation, your physician will be careful to screen for signs of development. It is not only important to share your family history, but also any signs or symptoms that you may be having. Never try to explain your way out of an unusual symptom. Instead always discuss such things with your physician, and allow them to be the one who determines the significance.

The Most Significant Genetic Red Lights

Determining your risk for developing inherited disorders can be quite complicated, and should be left to the medical professionals. However, there are a few genetic red lights that should make you run, not walk, to your annual exams. You say, what's the rush? The rush is that early detection is the best chance at a cure, or at least control, of the problem. If you wait too long, the best physician in the world cannot help you. Remember, physicians are not God, and miracles are nothing to be taken for granted.

Coronary Artery Disease (CAD) is a leading killer in both men and women, and often goes undetected or is ignored. Fortunately, we have the technology to detect early heart disease and reverse the pattern of damage. Genetically, many CAD disorders are linked to genes involved in the removal of LDL (low density lipoprotein), most commonly referred to as "bad Cholesterol." The inability to metabolize LDL can result in clogged arteries and many times death. Another form of CAD risk through genetic links has to do with the body's inability to clear homocysteine, a waste product found in the blood. There are two significant enzymes in the metabolism of homocysteine; the enzyme MTHFR, and Cystathione B-synthase (CBS). If mutation occurs in the genes that regulate these enzymes, heart disease is likely to develop.

Links between genetic mutations and blood pressure elevation are also being studied. It appears that a mutation called ACE (I/D) polymorphism may be responsible for the lack of regulation in blood pressure. More studies are being done to verify this correlation in larger populations.

Other genes, such as Apolipoprotein A1 (alpo A1) have been found to have mutations that lead to CAD. If there is a mutation in alpo A1, the body may have a decreased ability to produce high density lipoprotein (HDL), more commonly referred to as "good cholesterol." If the body is unable to produce sufficient levels of HDL, a person is more likely to have an early heart attack or stroke.

Colon Cancer has long been known to run in families in hereditary forms, such as familial adenomatous polyposis (FAP) and hereditary nonpolyposis colorectal cancer (HNPCC). Although the exact gene linkage has not been determined, each family member that has a history of colon cancer increases your risk of developing the disease in a significantly exponential way. For example, if one member of your family (parent or sibling) had colon cancer, you would be 1.7 times more likely to develop the disease. If two immediate relatives had cancer, your risk climbs to 2.7 times more likely to develop it.

Diabetes affects tens of millions of people in the developed world, and carries a stigma of being one of the leading causes of death. Early detection, and taking measures to gain control over the disease, is crucial in the overall outcome of those affected. While inherited genes play a large role in or chances for developing diabetes, the habits that we inherit are equally important. However, a combination of bad habits and bad genes is a sure sign of disaster. The genetic linkage for diabetes is complex, due to some mutations being cancelled out by other genetic factors. However, diabetes is closely related to obesity. The gene Beta3-Adrenergic Receptor makes a protein that is responsible for metabolism rates at rest. A mutation in this gene can lead to obesity, and therefore, an increased risk for type 2 diabetes.

Alzheimer's Disease is gaining more recognition, especially with the death of past president Ronald Reagan. Most people fear losing the function of their mental capacity more than anything. Alzheimer's disease is strongly linked to genetic mutation, and those who have a first-degree relative (parent or sibling) with the disease are at a 3.5 times greater risk for developing the disease. A mutation on the genes APP, PS1, or PS2 means a high likelihood of development of Alzheimer's. There are also other mutations of genes that are closely linked to the development of the disease.

Aging is inevitable, but one cannot help noticing the variance in the aging process. Genes have been identified and are being studied for their role in the aging process, as well as the changing molecular structure of the brain. In people that age rapidly, there has been a correlation in the expression of the genes related to stress, and inflammatory and immune responses. Although aging gracefully is a perk, not aging well is not necessarily a death sentence, just a quality of life issue. For some, that line is ill-defined.

Stopping the Train at the Station

Good health is never an accident, but instead a result of a conscious effort to take good care of one's body. Preventative measures and early detection are important in stopping problems before they get out of control. We have been blessed with the most advanced medical technology in the world, and healthcare is at its best. The possibilities for prevention are increasing daily, and the world of medicine is an exciting place to be. For our patients, it is a very lucky place to be. For those reading this book, you are perhaps the luckiest of all because such services are available and obtainable for you.

Coronary artery disease (CAD) is easier to detect than ever before. No longer are we dependent only upon assessing risk factors, such as high cholesterol and failed exercise stress tests. We are now able to incorporate actual images of the heart during an exercise stress test. This test is referred to as a thallium stress test and is becoming more widely available. As leaders in our field, we have the nuclear camera that the test requires right in our office. CAD is also detectable through coronary artery calcium scoring, which is done on a CT machine with special software that actually allows the physician to screen for plaque build-up on the arterial walls. Former President Clinton is an example to us all of the dangers of plaque build-up and the "ticking time bomb" that may be silently waiting to explode. Instead of taking drastic lifesaving measures during an emergency, CAD can be detected, and measures can be taken to reduce its level of significance. Although chest pain and shortness of breath may be present in CAD, it does not always carry warning signs. Screening for blockages and signs of the disease is a definite must of preventative medicine.

Colon cancer is many times discovered in its later stages. Rectal bleeding and other symptoms are often ignored or put off as hemorrhoids. All changes in bowel habits should be noted and discussed with your physician. Early detection of colon cancer significantly increases the survival rate. New technology allows for easy screening and early detection of colon cancers, and precancerous conditions. Through the use of software, a CAT scan of the abdomen can reconstruct the colon, and allow the physician to virtually "fly" through your colon on a computer screen and obtain 3D images. Polyps and cancer are easily identified, as well as the blood flow to such abnormalities. As a perk, our patients leave with a copy of their virtual colonoscopy on CD, thus allowing for hours of entertainment at home or at the office.

Type 2 diabetes can be detected early on if the patient is paying close attention to what their body is telling them. Symptoms such as excessive thirst or frequent urination are warning signs sometimes related to type 2 diabetes. These symptoms are often ignored by the patient. Simple blood test done in the office can detect the disease, and proper treatment measures can be taken. Often after a patient is diagnosed, weight loss and lifestyle management either decrease the significance of the problem or cure it all together. The key is to take good care of your body all the time, not just when you develop problems.

Alzheimer's disease is not curable, but early detection and intervention is important in slowing the disease process. Many physicians use mental capacity exams, also known as "mini mental status exams" or MMSE, to determine the likelihood of the disease, because until recently, only an autopsy could confirm the diagnosis. With the advancements of technology, Positron Emission Tomography (PET) Scans allow for early detection of the disease through the assessment of glucose metabolism in the brain. Early detection means early intervention. Ask anyone who has lost a loved one to Alzheimer's disease, and they will tell you that they would give anything to have one more day with that person. Even for those who struggle with the progression of the disease in a loved one, the loss of mental capacities is more than one should bear.

Aging, although somewhat linked to genetic predisposition, is often a matter of lifestyle choices. Choosing to exercise, eat right, and exercise the brain through continued stimulation and learning can help slow the aging process and increase your quality of life. Spending time in prayer or meditation has also been linked to longevity.

Taking ownership of your health is the best gift that you can give to yourself and your family. Having a handle on what risk factors you may posses, and dealing with those risk factors, can help optimize your chances for a longer, healthier life.

Chapter Six

The Executive Physical

Many times we are asked what makes the executive physical different from any other physical. There are multiple factors that contribute to the differences, but the main ones are time with the physician, and a thorough examination using the latest technology. Is the executive physical for everyone? It would be nice to offer this luxury to every person, but it is not practical. If you are lucky enough to be a patient of a clinic that practices executive medicine, you should expect the best in customer service, as well as top of the line medical care.

Taking Time with Your Physician

In the world of HMOs, medicine has become nothing more than patients being herded in like cattle to be seen in a sort of assembly line fashion. Fewer and fewer medical students are choosing to enter the field of primary care, and instead are opting for sub-specialties that see a lower volume at a higher reimbursement rate. Unfortunately, the person who suffers most is the patient. Patients desire and need more time with their physicians. The human race is becoming more complex, whereas we are living longer, and medical advancements allow us to detect and treat many illnesses early. Because of the shift in longevity, we should be getting just the opposite–more time, more thorough examination, and more advice.

The best way to obtain the needed time with a physician is to schedule it. Having a doctor that specializes in executive medicine, and practices low volume, high quality preventative medicine is well worth the investment. Just remember to be prepared to answer questions honestly and openly if you want to obtain the most benefit from your visit. All medical records and advice are confidential. Feeling embarrassed to ask questions and give the needed information is unwarranted.

Necessary Laboratory Tests

It is often necessary to run more than just the routine laboratory tests that are familiar to you. Laboratory advancements now allow for screening of many illnesses and diseases that once were considered "too late" when discovered. A list of laboratory tests and their purposes are listed below. This list is not all-inclusive, but will give you a better idea of what tests may be ordered and why. Not all of the tests listed will be a part of the executive physical.

The list is provided to give you a better understanding of the available technology.

- **Amylase**–Detects pancreatic inflammation.

- **Arthritis Panel**–Screens for lupus, rheumatoid arthritis, and other inflammatory diseases.

- **BNP**–Checks for heart failure.

- **Cardio C-Reactive Protein (Ultra-sensitive CRP)** –Detects inflammatory chemicals from blockages forming in the arteries of the body.

- **CA 125**–Cancer antigen count that helps detect ovarian tumors.

- **Complete Blood Count (CBC)**–Checks red and white blood cells, and platelets. This detects things such as leukemia, infection, and clotting disorders.

- **Comprehensive Metabolic Panel (CMP)**–Checks for electrolyte imbalances, kidney disorders, liver malfunction, protein status, and diabetes.

- **C-Reactive Protein (CRP)**–Marker of inflammation in the body.

- **Erythrocyte Sedimentation Rate (Sed Rate)**–Inflammatory marker.

• **Folic Acid Level**–Screens for a vitamin deficiency which is often related to anemia.

• **Follicular Stimulating Hormone (FSH)**–Pituitary hormone levels and menopause marker.

• **Glycosolated Hemoglobin (HGB A1C)**–Long-term measure of diabetic control.

• **Helicobacter Pylori**–Screens for a bacterial infection in the stomach that can be related to ulcers.

• **Hepatitis Panel**–Screens for hepatitis A, B, and C.

• **Hepatic Function Panel**–Screens for liver disease or inflammation.

• **Homocysteine Level**–Checks for progression of heart disease.

• **Lipid Panel (general)**–Checks cholesterol (HDL and LDL) and triglycerides.

• **Lipid Panel (advanced)**–In addition to the general lipid panel, checks for particle size, which is related to blockage in the arteries.

• **PAP Smear (preferably Thin Prep®)**–Screens for cervical cancer and inflammation.

• **Partial Thromboplastin Time (PTT)**–Checks clotting ability.
• **Prolactin**–Pituitary hormone deficiency that can cause loss of libido, or breast discharge in women.

• **Prothrombin Time (PT with INR)**–Checks clotting ability.

• **Stool for Occult Blood**–Screens for blood in the stool that may indicate colon cancer, inflammatory disease of the bowel, diverticulosis, or bleeding polyps.

• **Testosterone (total and free)**–Screens for testosterone deficiency which may cause impotence or loss of muscle mass.

• **Thyroid Stimulating Hormone (TSH)**–Screens for thyroid dysfunction.

• **Urinalysis**–Urine screening for infection and renal function.

• **Vitamin B12 levels**–Screen for vitamin deficiency often related to fatigue and pernicious anemia.

Imaging for Early Detection

It is amazing to us as physicians to see all the medical advancements that have taken place, especially in imaging, over the last decade. We are so blessed as Americans to have the technology readily available to detect abnormalities, and often prevent problems from becoming fatal. Even when life-threatening discoveries are made, we have a better chance at beating the odds than ever before. Different types of imaging are discussed in this chapter, but all are not routine for the executive physical.

Computed Axial Tomography (CAT or CT Scan)

In the early 1970s, Godfrey Hounsfield of EMI Laboratories in England invented the first CAT scan machine. By the early 1980s, these machines were integrated into mainstream medicine. Over the years, the technology of the CAT scan machine has advanced exponentially and is now used to identify numerous abnormalities.

A CAT scan works by visualizing parts of the body in 3-D, rather than the traditional 2-D x-ray. Because the images are in 3-D format, tumors and other abnormalities can be easily identified. A CAT scan machine obtains pictures and allows the radiologist to view the images in slices. This way of viewing makes it very difficult for abnormalities to hide deep within organs without detection. With the advancements of technology, the CAT scan takes only a matter of seconds to obtain numerous images.

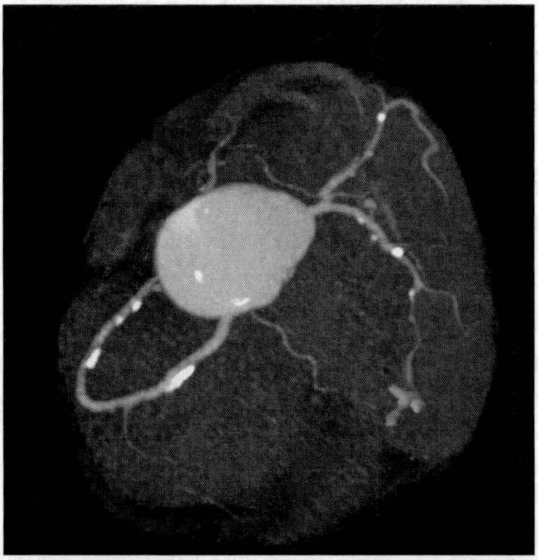

This CT of the coronary arteries shows blockages that can cause heart attacks (shown here as white spots).

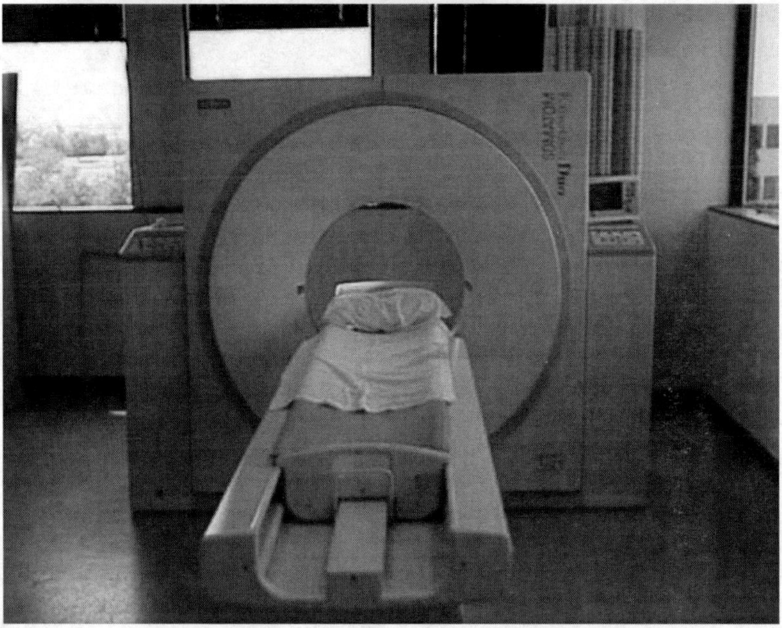

GE Light Speed Pro Cat Scan Machine.
Photo courtesy of Healthcare Associates of Irving.

A partial list of uses for the CAT scan machine is listed below:

- **Calcium Scoring of the Coronary Arteries**–Identifies plaque build-up in the arteries and detect coronary artery disease in its earliest stages.

- **CT of Abdomen/Pelvis**–Used to identify organ tumors, inflammation, malfunction, and other abnormalities.

- **CT of Chest**–Identifies cancer, benign tumors, asbestosis, and other lung and chest cavity abnormalities.

- **CT of Head**–Used to identify brain tumors, aneurysms, strokes, and many other problems.

- **CTA of the Coronary Arteries**–This procedure allows clear images that were once only possible through catheterization of these arteries. As technology is advancing, it is believed that catheterization will become obsolete, and the images through CTA will soon be gold standard for detecting blockages.

- **CTA of Other Arteries**–Blockage detection in the peripheral arteries and carotid arteries can now be viewed through CTA with the same clarification of catheterization.

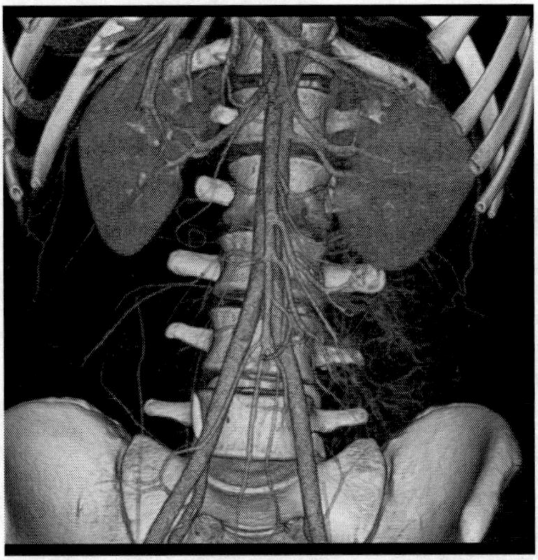

This is a CTA image of renal arteries.
Photo courtesy of Healthcare Associates of Irving.

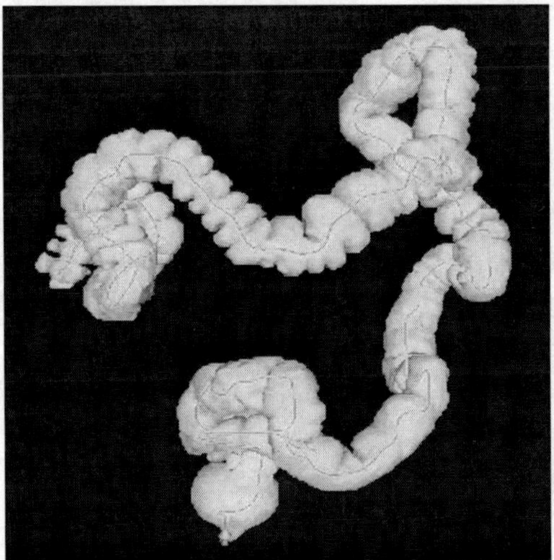

Software, such as Viatronix®, allows for CT 3-D reconstruction of the colon. This procedure is also referred to as virtual colonoscopy.

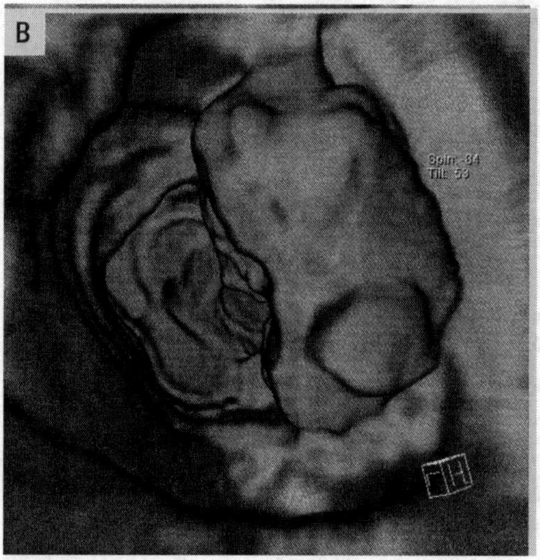

This image is of a colon cancer found by a virtual colonoscopy procedure.

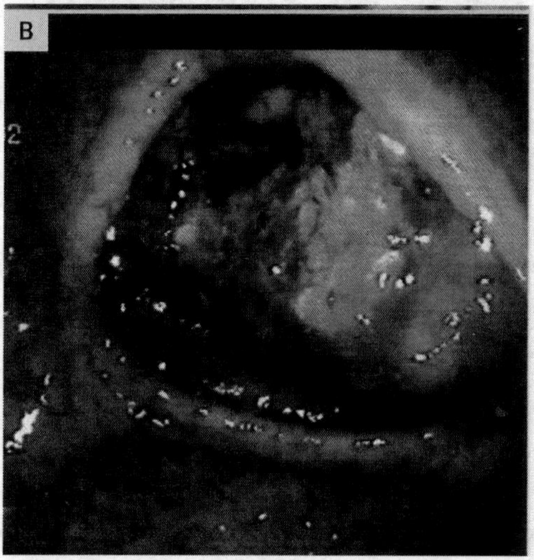

The same tumor is shown here with a optical colnocopy prior to surgery.

• **Virtual Colonoscopy**–Uses CT technology to reconstruct the colon in 3-D and identify polyps (pre-cancer), colon cancer, inflammatory bowel diseases, internal hemorrhoids, Crohn's Disease and other colon abnormalities.

• **DEXA (Dual Energy X-ray Absortiometry) Scan** Osteoporosis is a serious condition in which the bones become brittle and break easily. With the use of a DEXA scan, osteoporosis can be diagnosed, and treatment can be given to stop the progression of the deterioration. In some cases, the patient may be able to take medication that helps to strengthen the existing bone. This procedure should be a part of the executive physical for women who are over the age of 40, or who have a family history of osteoporosis.

Osteoporosis Facts

- In the U.S. today, 10 million individuals are estimated to already have the disease and almost 34 million more are estimated to have low bone mass, placing them at increased risk for osteoporosis.
- Of the 10 million Americans estimated to have osteoporosis, eight million are women and 2 million are men.
- Thirty-four million Americans have low bone mass, which puts them at increased risk of developing osteoporosis and related fractures.
- One in two women and one in four men over age 50 will have an osteoporosis-related fracture in her/his remaining lifetime.

Source: National Osteoporosis Foundation

• Magnetic Resonance Imaging (MRI)

The beginning phases of what we now know as MRI started in 1946, when Felix Bloch and Edward Purcell both independently discovered the magnetic resonance phenomenon. They both won the Nobel Prize in 1952 for their discoveries. However, it was not until the 1970's that Raymond Damadian found a way to use the technology for medical imaging of the human body. Today, the hard work of these brilliant scientists is responsible for saving millions of lives and paving the way for other medical advancements.

MRI is a widely used imaging technique in which the human body can be imaged and viewed in either 2-D or 3-D. The machine uses a giant magnet, unlike x-ray and CT scanners that use radiation. The technology of the MRI allows for identification of different tissue abnormalities as well as injury assessment. MRI is often used as a tool to guide surgeons prior to surgery, since it can pinpoint the problem and identify the major issues.

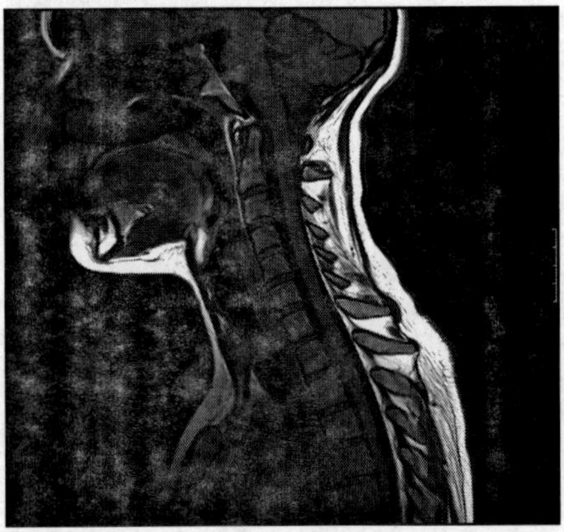

This MRI of the spine shows the cervical disks clearly and makes it easy to diagnose any problems. Photo courtesy of Siemens Medical Solutions.

Some types of MRI scans are listed below:

• **MRI of the Head**–Can identify tumors, multiple sclerosis, aneurysms, strokes, and other neurological abnormalities.

• **MRI of the Knee**–Identifies injuries to the knee that may not be identifiable on x-ray, such as tendon and muscle injuries.

• **MRI of the Shoulder**–This is usually performed if there has been an injury to the shoulder that has limited the range of motion. It can determine the best course of action–surgery or physical therapy.

• **MRI of the Spine**–Identifies injuries to the c-spine (neck), T-spine (mid back), or LS-spine (lower back), such as disc injuries or deterioration. MRI scans of the head may also be ordered with a MRA (Magnetic Resonance Angiography). MRA allows the blood vessels of the brain to be viewed without the need for contrast.

Nuclear Medicine

The mid 1930s boast of the discovery of "artificial radioactivity." This advancement is linked to the success of nuclear medicine today. In 1946, a fascinating discovery was made when a patient with thyroid cancer was cured with radioactive iodine. Since that time, the use of nuclear medicine in clinical settings has compounded. Nuclear medicine is now used in many applications; the most recent is the detection of heart disease.

This Nuclear Camera is part of the Siemens Signature Series. Photo courtesy of Executive Medicine of Southlake

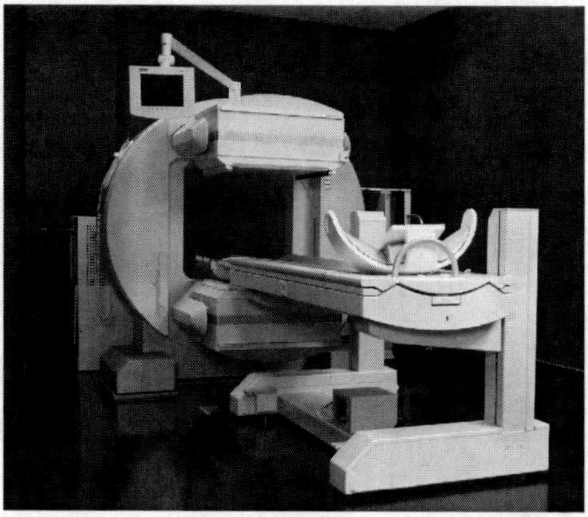

A partial list of nuclear testing is found below:

• **Adenosine Scan**–Allows the heart to be chemically stimulated and, can be done in place of the thallium stress test in patients who can not perform the tread-mill tests.

• **Bone Scan**–Can be whole body or regional scans that identify bone cancers and other abnormalities.

• **HIDA**–Scans the gallbladder for stones and bile duct abnormalities.

• **Thallium Stress Test**–Combines the traditional treadmill test with nuclear medicine to allow for not only tracings, but also actual images of the heart at work. This is becoming the gold standard for heart disease detection because it catches blockages more readily than traditional methods alone.

• **Thyroid Scan with Uptake**–Identifies thyroid function and size.

• **Positron Emission Tomography (PET) Scan**
The PET scanner, which was used in the 70s and 80s primarily for research, made its way into hospitals and imaging centers in the 1990s as a way to detect cancer and monitor therapy progress. In the 2000s, PET has shown to also be a promising diagnostic tool for Alzheimer's disease, catching the disease many times before symptoms surface. PET technology is now being used to track brain disorders and heart tissue damage.

Unlike the CT or MRI, the PET tracks the biological changes of tissue. It not only identifies tumors, but can actually determine the type of tumor based on cellular activity. During a PET exam, an injection of a radioactive substance is given to the patient, and then the body is scanned to obtain images of the area in question. If the scan is being performed to determine a cancer diagnosis or track the progress of cancer treatment, the biological make-up of the tumor can be examined. If the scan is being performed for heart disease, the results can determine if a person has had a heart attack. Combined with a cardiac perfusion study, it can be determined if any of the tissue is damaged, and if blood flow is being restricted. In Alzheimer's disease, the metabolism of glucose in the brain can be tracked and the disease can be caught in the earliest of stages.

PET scan is becoming a fast growing tool for physicians to use when diagnosing a patient. It is a prime example of how fortunate we are to live in an age of medical technology unseen by our ancestors. Such technology is also a precursor to what lies ahead for the next generation.

Lifestyle Assessment and Management

Absolutely no executive level physical is complete without a thorough lifestyle assessment. The assessment should cover questions about your general health, eating habits, exercise habits, smoking history, work environment history, stress levels, and much more. It is very important to get a glimpse at the big picture of one's lifestyle, and thoroughly explore the pitfalls and the triumphs, prior to making suggestions on how to manage things in the future.

Failing to assess the lifestyle of an individual is equivalent to going for a check-up on your car and ignoring the oil, a basic necessity. Lifestyles of individuals can vary in so many degrees. You may travel more than most, or follow a vegetarian diet; whereas, others may stay close to home and have meat and potatoes each night for dinner. Each individual has unique needs. Your physician should be able to key into those needs, and help you to develop a plan of action for meeting them while increasing your overall health.

Fitness Assessment

Sometimes people who hear the words "fitness assessment" immediately think of a gym and lifting weights. While that is one way to obtain fitness, for the sake of a physical exam, we are more interested in the overall fitness level of an individual. Finding out what the current exercise regiment is will help determine if more is needed, or if the current plan needs to be modified. Exercise is hard on the body, and not everyone should exercise in the same manner. By tying the physical exam in with the fitness assessment, the individual is given a plan that is safe and effective for their physical condition, backed by their physician's stamp of approval.

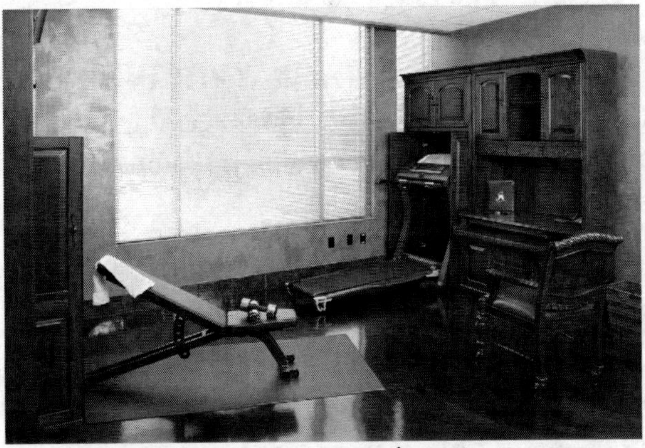

Fitness Assessments are an important part of executive physicals. Photo courtesy of Executive Medicine of Southlake

DNA Analysis

The advancements in DNA analysis have been one of the most interesting and complex discoveries of our time. Although much information can come from DNA analysis, we will focus in on the types of testing that can be done, and should be done, as part of an executive physical. Below is a list of tests that are important in determining the proper preventative medicine regiment for an individual.

• **Bone Health Gene (BH-2, COL1A1)**: This gene is responsible for the production of protein that is important to bone growth and health.

• **Detoxification (METHX)**: These genes are important in detoxifying the body from environmental pollutants, such as cigarette smoke and exhaust from automobiles and machinery.

• **Heart Circulatory Health -1 (HCH-1, PON-1)**: This gene helps prevent blockage due to plaque build-up on blood vessel walls. It is important in the prevention of heart disease.

• **Heart Circulatory Health–2 (HCH-2, MTHFR)**: This gene helps prevent the build-up of homocysteine. If levels of homocysteine are high, there is a risk for higher cholesterol, increased risk for blood clots, and damage to blood vessels.

• **Immune Gene (IM-1, TNF-A)**: This gene is important to proper immune responses and signals immune cells to areas that are in need of the healing process.

• **Oxidative Stress 1 (OS-1Gene, MNSOD)**: This gene is important in protecting the body against oxidative stress and wards off free radical molecules.

• **Oxidative Stress 2 (OS-2 Gene, GTX1)**: This gene is important in detoxifying hydrogen peroxide, one of the molecules that will form during oxidative stress and damage good cells.

These DNA tests can be done through a simple cheek swab and will take a few weeks for results. The results are very important when determining preventative measures, especially vitamin supplementation for an individual. Since not every person has the same needs, obtaining the proper regiment will ensure that you can live up to your optimum health and perform at peak levels.

Vitamin Supplementation

Just as each individual is different, so is his or her vitamin supplementation needs. Needs are dependant on lifestyle, dietary regiments, and as noted above, DNA findings. At one time, we told everyone to take a multivitamin that was easily found at any drug store. Since then, we have realized that individuals have different needs. Not only are deficiency levels different, but taking too much of a vitamin that may already be adequately met through one's diet can be harmful. For example, taking an excess of anti-oxidants can be counter productive because it may cause a slow in metabolic processes. Vitamin supplements are not all the same, and asking every individual to take the same regiment is not practical, nor is it good preventative medicine.

Chapter Seven

Maintenance

It is always interesting to see how well people will take care of their cars, insist that their lawns are nicely manicured, and do the proper upkeep on their homes. It is an unfortunate fact that most people do not go to such lengths to maintain their health: Especially when all the necessities and extras are dependent on a person's ability to function. No matter how much you have invested in your properties, your most important investment is you and your health.

Yearly Physical: 365-Mile Maintenance Plan

While it is recommended that different age groups obtain physicals either on a yearly, every two year, or every five year schedule dependent on age, we recommend that executives have a physical each year regardless of age. Because executives have high levels of stress, spend many hours traveling, tend to eat out frequently, and work long hours and at high mental capacity, it is best to keep abreast of their overall health. A good comparison is the maintenance on a high performance car. One would never drive a high performance car at peak performance, day in and day out, without getting the proper maintenance. Therefore, you can think of your yearly physical as a 365-mile maintenance plan for your body, which is used to optimize peak performance, check the liquid levels, tune up the transmission, and review all diagnostic testing results. Only thing is–you are worth far more than the most expensive car available.

Keeping Good Records

Any physician, no matter how skilled, can only gather the whole picture of your health with your cooperation. You must keep good records. Telling your physician that you had a pain somewhere, you can not remember where, and you are not sure how long it lasted, is useless. Instead, keep copious notes on important changes in your body. If you have unexplained pains, change in mood, change in eating habits, decreased energy levels, sleep disturbances, or a change in bowel habits, let your physician know. In many cases, do not wait until your physical exam if it is more than a month away. Things such as chest pain, shortness of breath, blood in the stool, or visual changes should be reported immediately.

It may be best to follow a chart of some sort, and for this reason, a chart has been created in the

Appendix A for you to use. Keeping good records will not only make you aware of your health, but will allow your physician to assess your complaints and make proper diagnoses.

Following Advice

Let's face it, if you were not interested in optimizing your health, you would not be sitting here reading this book. Therefore, when you obtain your physical examination and recommendations, it is important that you follow the advice that your physician has provided. Using the car analogy, you would probably never dream of putting regular gas in the tank of a high performance tank that calls for high-octane fuel only; and if you did, the results would eventually be devastating. Taking short cuts or making cheap substitutions for your high performance body is equally damaging.

A good executive physical will breakdown your overall health assessment and give good, sound advice that is easy to follow. Following that advice will help you to live healthier, obtain optimal mental capacity, and contribute to a more balanced lifestyle.

Chapter Eight

Defining 100%

It is often said that we should give 100% at everything we do. This is something that we have heard all of our lives. Every test we have ever taken is marked by 100% for perfection, and even the juice boxes we buy for our children brag of 100% juice. We all have an idea of what it all means, but when it comes to life, we are not sure how to apply it in a way that is obtainable.

In a mathematical equation, if you have 100% of something, it becomes whole or complete. If you have less, let's say 88%, there is a 12% gap from the optimum level. The same is true for yourself, home, work, and children. Giving 100% to each of them seems impossible, especially since mathematically that would equal 400%. It is a matter of priorities, and you should give 100% of your devoted time to the priority at hand. When you move on to the next priority, focus on it alone and again give 100%. Thinking of how to structure a business deal while playing T-ball with little Tommy does not allow for either to have 100% of your focus. The end result is added stress and disorganized thoughts.

Prioritizing

As a way to make your day less hectic and much more fulfilled, prioritizing must happen. Each of us only has 24 hours in a day, no more, no less. How we choose to spend our 24 hours is up to us. One option is to wake up and let the day take you for a ride. Answer calls while you are trying to meet other deadlines, weed through the interruptions, and when you get home, try to make sense of it all as the day replays through your head once more. Obviously, this is not the best option. All day long, you would have given 10–90% of your attention to each thing, while thinking about something else. Even though you can get some things accomplished, it is not the best option for success or personal satisfaction.

Instead of choosing option one, let's take another look at how our day could go. First, you get up and spend 100% of your first thirty minutes with your spouse, or just relaxing with the paper. Then, you drive or commute to work, taking this time to mentally prepare for the day. While at the office, you ask for no interruptions as you tackle the task at hand with 100% of your efforts and focus. Around lunch, you check in with the family and then enjoy your meal, hopefully a healthy one. After you eat, you return calls and handle the things that are urgent, giving 100% of your attention to the details, and reaching as many conclusions on those problems as possible. From, say two o'clock on, you get back to the task at hand and give 100% of your attention to the project. Since you did not finish, you quickly jot down notes of where to pick up tomorrow and at what time you should complete what is left. Now, you take the last thirty minutes of the day devoting 100% of your attention on your employees. Take a moment to ask them how their day was, if they need anything, and maybe throw in a few anecdotes that will end the day on an upbeat note.

The day is not over at five o'clock, as most of us know. If you have a family at home, only phase two begins at this point. If you have stayed focused all day, you will have the ability to continue 100% until you retire for the night. At this point you are on your way home from the office, and you should be either spending 100% of your time listening to music you like, or resetting your brain (as we discussed in an earlier chapter). This will allow you to accept those at home with open arms. This is where it gets tricky, because you are taking off your business hat and replacing it with your spouse hat, and/or Dad or Mom hat. You must remember that the big powerful executive has left the office, and is headed home to those loved ones. If you are not married or have kids, this is where you take time to foster the friendships and relationships you do have, or to make more.

Wearing the home hats is not always easy because they, unlike the corporate world, do not come with Standard Operating Procedures (SOPs).

Instead, it is up to you to put in effort and use your best judgment to handle things. We all wish that universities offered degrees in marriage and parenting, but such degrees simply do not exist. Your kids are not perfect, and neither is your spouse, nor are you for that matter. No matter what your spouse does for a living, or if they stay at home, always remember the following tips:

•Be humble; do not compare your day with theirs. Yes, you have worked hard, but you have no idea what their day was like.

•Do not spend all your time talking about the office. A few stories, if asked, will suffice. Do not let your family feel like they are second fiddle. If you spend too much time reminiscing about your day at the office, you are not going to be able to give 100% attention where it is now needed.

•Be upfront with your family. There are times that you need to give 100% to yourself, even if it is only thirty minutes a day. Remember, they will need to do the same.

•Spend time with your children asking them about their day. This is not a time to lecture them on success and learning from mistakes. Simply listen. The more you listen, the more they will talk.

•Always say good night to everyone in the house.

Never go off to bed without a good night ritual. If you have forgotten how to do this, try to catch a re-run of The Walton's.

These tips are just the beginning, and there are many other great tips found in self-help books. One of the best books that is often recommended in marriage counseling, and to all our married couples, is "*His Needs Her Needs: Building an Affair-Proof Marriage*" by Willard F. Harley, Jr. Even if you think you are the best spouse to walk the face of this earth and your marriage is great, read it anyway.

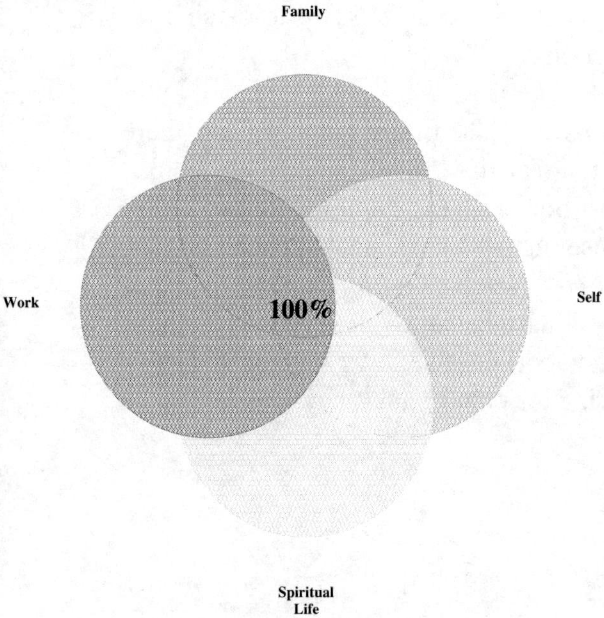

When aspects of life constantly beg for attention, they only stea from each other. This pattern creates chaos from the mental and emotional overlap.

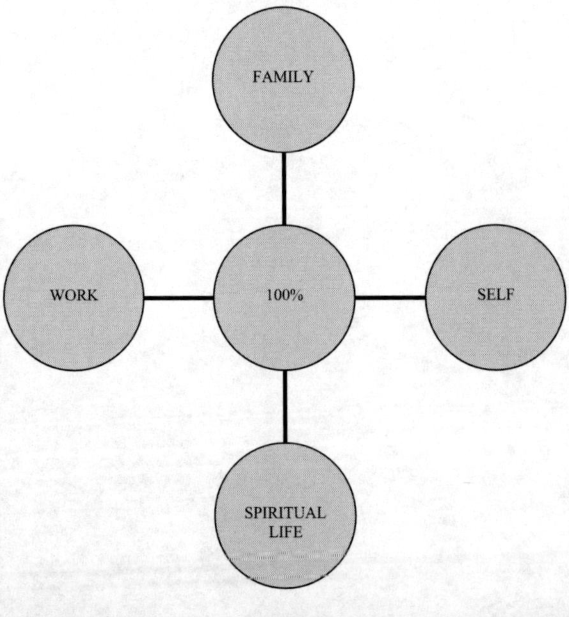

This diagram is a demonstratio of how each aspect of life should be considered a separate entity. Individual attention is important if one wishes to obtain well rounded aspects of their life.

Executive Coaching

Executive coaching is becoming more and more popular among the leaders of top companies and the owners of successful small businesses. It teaches how to obtain the 100% goal. We are not born with the ability to tackle complex problems and make business decisions. Even the best business schools in the country cannot prepare you for everything that will come your way. It is doubtful that any school in the country teaches how to balance our successful lives at work with our hopefully successful home life. As a matter of fact, it is no secret that the most successful people at work have home lives that have a lot to be desired, and vice versa.

As part of our research, we sought out one of the nation's top executive coaches, Rachna D. Jain, PsyD, owner of Excel With Ease International, LLC. Her website is www.excelwitheasecoaching.com. She is published, has a degree in Psychology, is a Certified Comprehensive Coach, and is well respected among her peers. Although you may have seen her quoted in such places as the *Washington Post* and the *Ladies Home Journal,* Dr. Jain has also had the honor of coaching some of today's top executives. An interview with her included below, as a way to better help you understand the benefits of executive coaching.

Q. What is executive coaching?

Executive Coaching is the process of an executive becoming better at their job and creating more life satisfaction. Coaching includes stress management, skills building (especially communication), time management, and finding balance. Executives who are coached and apply the new skills tend to take better care of themselves, become more organized, obtain balance in their life, find boundaries, and are able to correct bad habits and develop good ones. Executive coaching helps people pull out of the ditch and get moving again.

Q. When did executive coaching become popular?

The traditional informal level of mentoring among colleagues has dwindled due to time constraints and competitiveness. People have turned to coaching because when using a coach, ideas can be bounced off the coach without the fear of rejection or loss of respect. In the early 1990's, it became more popular to seek advice in a workshop. Now, through executive coaching, advice is more personalized to the individual and the type of work they do. Not only are larger companies enjoying the benefits of the executives that have been coached, but small business owners are reaping benefits of their own personal gains through coaching.

Q. How can executive coaching improve health and quality of life?

Executive coaching gives practical applications in making clarifications for change, and the support to make those changes. Some of the techniques used include role playing, journaling, and developing different responses to stressors. Executive coaches offer social support, but also make you take personal responsibility for your health. Not only does the coach help the person make strides toward better personal health, they encourage healthier relationships with loved ones and employees. As an executive coach, I discourage martyring and instead help instill a strong sense of confidence. Such confidence has to come from deep inside and no longer from the outside and artificial. Basically, with executive coaching, the mountains disappear, and they simply become bumps in the road.

Q. Who are the best candidates for executive coaching?

Everyone could benefit from executive coaching, although the best clients are the ones who try to change, because they have insight into the fact that the current situation is not working. The client must have the commitment to change for the better and the patience to see the process through. Although most executives like to delegate, this is the one thing that cannot be delegated and they must do themselves.

Q. What should one look for in an executive coach?

First, they should be credentialed. Next, the client must feel a level of comfort with their coach, and have the added reassurance that the coach they choose has experience with clients in similar situations or professions. If you are seeking a coach, you should also make sure that the availability of the coach meets your schedule.

Anytime you interview, you usually speak to more than one person. The same holds true when finding an executive coach. Interview at least three until you find the right one for you.

Q. How much time is involved in the executive coaching process?

Coaching should take place for at least 3 consecutive months. Pattern changing takes time and practice. Therefore, the client must be willing to work at the process outside of the scheduled session by applying what they have learned and analyzing the results. With every change in life, the participant must be willing to conform to new ideas and apply the new techniques.

Q. What is the financial investment that one can expect?

It all depends on the scope of work, but $3,000-$10,000 is an expected range. However, if the person applies the techniques learned, the return on investment can be far above the initial expense.

Q. Is there anything else you would like to add?

Yes. Although the executive coaching applies

to both men and women, I always like to share an interesting fact that I learned: Married men live longer than unmarried men, and happily married men live longer that unhappily married men.

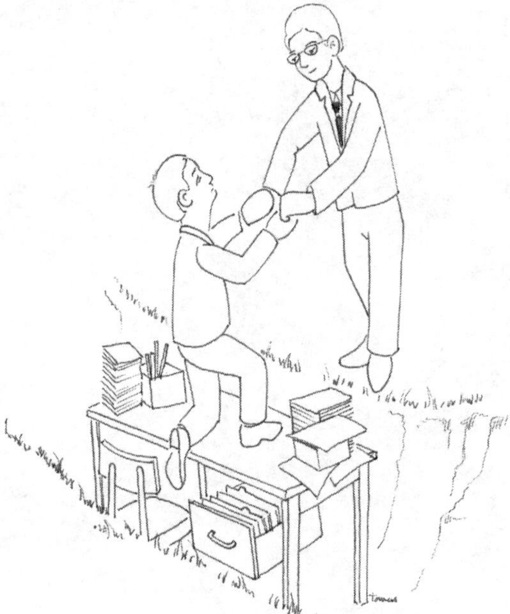

Executive Coaches can lift you out of the trenches.

CHAPTER NINE

TYING IT ALL TOGETHER

As leaders in the medical field, it is our duty to give sound advice on how you can obtain optimal health. As the health needs of busy executives become more noticed, we will have laid the ground for meeting those needs. This book has given you a brief history of medicine and how we arrived at where we are today, as well as covered many important aspects of executive health and preventative measures. Taking care of the body that God has blessed you with, and protecting your mental capacities is not only important, it is your responsibility. You have a responsibility to your Creator, your family, and yourself, to get in and stay in the best health possible.

Below is a checklist of some of the main points covered in the book. Look over the list and see where you have needs for improvement.

- Do I have a clear understanding of the stressors, both physically and mentally, that I face each day?

- Am I paying attention to my nutritional needs?

• Do I travel in a way that ensures the least amount of stress on my body as possible?

• How am I handling my home and work life? Is there balance? What would my spouse say?

• Do I have my own personal space? Is my space conducive to my need for relaxation?

• Do I know my family history?

• What are my genetic predispositions?

• Am I taking proper preventative measures to ward off diseases and disorders that I may genetically be predisposed?

• Am I making sure that I have a physical exam yearly?

• Is my physical exam on the level of those described in this book? (Is it a 365-mile maintenance plan or just an oil check?)

• Am I keeping good records of my health and any possible problems?

• Do I follow medical advice?

• Do I understand what 100% is?

• Am I giving 100% in each area of my life?

• Could I benefit from executive coaching?

• How would I rate my overall health on a scale of 1–10?

• Am I taking personal responsibility for the optimization of my health?

In your journey through life, take time to take good care of your body, mind, and spirit. This book is just the beginning of your road ahead. Best wishes.